PEPTIC ULCER DIET COOKBOOK

Meal Plans And Healing Recipes To Soothe Stomach Pain, Reduce Acid Reflux, And Promote Digestive Health

DR ELIAN GRIFFIN

Copyright © [Elian Griffin] [2024]. All rights reserved.

Without the publisher's prior written consent, no portion of this publication may be copied, distributed, or transmitted in any way, including by photocopying, recording, or other mechanical or electronic means, with the exception of brief quotations used in all critical reviews.

DISCLAIMER

The nutritional recommendations and recipes in this book are meant solely for informative reasons. They are not meant to replace the counsel, diagnosis, or care of a qualified medical expert. If you have any doubts about a medical condition or dietary requirements, you should always see your physician or another trained healthcare expert.

All reasonable efforts have been taken by the author and publisher to ensure that the information contained in this book is correct as of the date of publication. Recommendations may alter, though, as medical knowledge is always changing. When using any of the recipes or instructions found here, the user assumes all liability and assumes no risk, whether personal or otherwise. People who have certain dietary requirements or medical issues should speak with a healthcare provider for personalized guidance. The given recipes are only ideas; you may need to adjust them to suit your own nutritional needs, tastes, and tolerances.

When you use this book, you agree to release the publisher, the author, and their representatives from any liability for any claims, damages, liabilities, costs, or expenditures resulting from your use of the book.

TABLE OF CONTENTS

CHAPTER ONE 11
PEPTIC ULCER DIET INTRODUCTION 11
- COMPREHENDING PEPTIC ULCERS 11
- DIET IS CRUCIAL FOR MANAGING PEPTIC ULCERS 12
- HOW THIS COOKBOOK CAN BE USEFUL 13
- ADVICE ON HOW TO USE THIS COOKBOOK 14
- FAQS & FREQUENTLY ASKED QUESTIONS 15

CHAPTER TWO 17
AN OVERVIEW OF PEPTIC ULCERS 17
- HOW DO PEPTIC ULCERS OCCUR? 17
- PEPTIC ULCER CAUSES 17
- SIGNS AND PROGNOSIS 18
- PEPTIC ULCER TYPES 19
- DIET IS IMPORTANT FOR TREATMENT 20

CHAPTER THREE 21
FUNDAMENTALS OF A DIET FOR PEPTIC ULCERS 21
- OBJECTIVES OF THE DIET 21
- FOODS TO ADD 22
- FOOD TO AVOID 23
- TIPS FOR MEAL PLANNING 23
- ESSENTIALS FOR THE PANTRY AND SHOPPING 24

CHAPTER FOUR 27
MEAL PLANNING AND PREPARATION 27
- WEEKLY MEAL PLANNING SCHEDULE 27

STRATEGIES FOR BATCH COOKING 28

ADVICE FOR DINING OUT 30

RECIPES FOR OPTIMAL DIGESTIVE HEALTH 31

EASY COOKING USING KITCHEN TOOLS 32

RECIPES FOR BREAKFAST 34

    HEALTHY DRINKS 34

    FIBER-PACKED OATMEAL CONVERSIONS 35

    WHOLESOME EGG RECIPES 36

    LOW-ACID FRUIT SELECTIONS 37

    IDEAS FOR QUICK AND SIMPLE BREAKFASTS 38

RECIPES FOR LUNCH 40

    LIGHT DRESSINGS AND SALADS 40

    OPTIONS FOR LEAN PROTEIN 41

    WHOLE GRAIN SELECTIONS 42

    VEGETABLE-BASED RECIPES 43

    IDEAS FOR CARRYING LUNCH ON THE GO 44

RECIPES FOR DINNER 45

    DELICIOUS FISH AND SHELLFISH 45

    ENTREES WITH LEAN MEAT 46

    MAIN COURSES FOR VEGETARIANS 47

    ASSORTMENTS AND SIDE DISHES 48

    ONE-POT DINNER IDEAS 49

RECIPES FOR SNACKS AND DESSERTS 50

    HEALTHY SNACK SUGGESTIONS 50

    YOGURT AND FRESH FRUIT PARFAITS 51

- LOW-CARB BAKED GOODS 52
- SWEETS WITH VERY LITTLE SUGAR 53
- TIPS FOR HEALTHY SNACKING 54
- DRINKS AND SMOOTHIES 56
  - OPTIONS FOR HYDRATING DRINKS 56
  - RECIPES FOR ANTI-INFLAMMATORY SMOOTHIES 57
  - HERBAL INFUSIONS AND TEAS 58
  - A LOOK AT COFFEE AND CAFFEINE 59
  - THE EFFECTS OF ALCOHOL 60
- CHAPTER FIVE 61
  - RECIPES FOR SPECIAL OCCASIONS AND HOLIDAYS 61
    - IDEAS FOR HOLIDAY MEALS 61
    - INGREDIENTS THAT ARE IN SEASON 62
    - TIPS FOR GUESTS WITH PEPTIC ULCERS 62
    - MODIFYING RECIPES FOR EVENTS 63
- CHAPTER SIX 65
  - TIPS FOR STRESS MANAGEMENT AND LIFESTYLE 65
    - STRESS MANAGEMENT'S SIGNIFICANCE 65
    - TECHNIQUES FOR RELAXATION 66
    - EXERCISE FOR A HEALTHY DIGESTIVE SYSTEM 68
    - THE FUNCTION OF SLEEP 69
    - MODIFICATIONS TO LIFESTYLE FOR EXTENDED WELL-BEING 70

ABOUT THE BOOK

Peptic ulcers are characterized by painful sores in the lining of the stomach or upper part of the small intestine. Peptic ulcers require careful attention to diet to alleviate symptoms and promote healing. The Peptic Ulcer Diet Cookbook is an invaluable resource for anyone managing peptic ulcers, providing a comprehensive approach to dietary management and overall wellness. It is important to understand the basics of peptic ulcers, including their causes, symptoms, diagnosis, and different types, which this book thoroughly explains to arm readers with vital knowledge.

A customized diet that promotes healing and reduces discomfort is essential to managing peptic ulcers. This cookbook explains the fundamentals of a peptic ulcer diet, with an emphasis on objectives like lowering acidity and irritation while improving digestive health. It offers precise instructions on which foods to include because of their healing qualities and which ones to avoid because they can worsen symptoms. It also includes helpful meal planning advice and pantry essentials to make it simple for readers to implement these dietary guidelines into their daily lives and ensure sustained adherence for long-term relief.

The cookbook is organized into chapters that address different meal times and occasions and provide a variety of recipes that are healthy and geared toward digestive health. For example, each chapter includes balanced recipes for lunch and dinner that include lean proteins, whole grains, and vegetable-focused dishes, as well as snack and dessert ideas, hydrating beverages, and recipes for special occasions. All of these things ensure that people with peptic ulcers can still enjoy a wide variety of delicious meals without sacrificing their health goals.

Beyond recipes, the book answers frequently asked questions and provides helpful guidance on meal planning, dining out, and stress management—factors that can have a big impact on managing ulcers.

Lifestyle modifications, such as stress reduction practices, relaxation techniques, and appropriate exercise regimens, are also highlighted to support overall digestive wellness and maximize the effectiveness of dietary changes.

Essentially, the "Peptic Ulcer Diet Cookbook" is more than just a cookbook; it's an all-encompassing guide that enables people to take charge of their health by making educated dietary decisions and adopting a more holistic lifestyle. Through the integration of professional advice with doable tactics, this cookbook promotes healing as well as a long-term, sustainable method of treating peptic ulcers.

CHAPTER ONE

PEPTIC ULCER DIET INTRODUCTION

COMPREHENDING PEPTIC ULCERS

The lining of the stomach, small intestine, or esophagus can become sore from peptic ulcers, which are typically caused by the erosion of the protective mucus layer that normally shields these tissues from the acidic digestive juices. Common symptoms include heartburn, nausea, vomiting, and burning stomach pain. Effective management requires an understanding of the underlying causes, which can include Helicobacter pylori infection, chronic use of nonsteroidal anti-inflammatory drugs (NSAIDs), excessive alcohol consumption, and smoking.

Understanding these factors is essential to effectively managing and alleviating symptoms associated with peptic ulcers. To diagnose peptic ulcers, doctors typically perform an endoscopy or other imaging tests to visualize the ulcerated areas.

Treatment aims to promote healing of the ulcerated tissues and reduce acid production in the stomach. This often involves medications such as proton pump inhibitors (PPIs) to reduce stomach acid and antibiotics to eradicate H. pylori infections if present. Lifestyle changes, including stress management and avoiding NSAIDs and alcohol, are also recommended to prevent ulcer recurrence.

DIET IS CRUCIAL FOR MANAGING PEPTIC ULCERS

A well-balanced diet can help minimize symptoms and prevent complications associated with peptic ulcers. Key dietary principles include consuming foods that are low in acidity and fat to minimize irritation to the stomach lining.

It's also important to avoid spicy foods, caffeine, and alcohol, as these can exacerbate symptoms and increase stomach acid production. Diet plays a crucial role in managing peptic ulcers by helping to reduce stomach acid production and promote healing of the ulcerated tissues.

Following these dietary guidelines can help individuals manage peptic ulcers and improve their overall digestive health. Other helpful foods to include in your diet include oatmeal, yogurt, bananas, and honey.

Eating smaller, more frequent meals throughout the day instead of large ones can also help manage symptoms by reducing the workload on the stomach. Finally, drinking plenty of water and avoiding carbonated beverages is essential to maintaining stomach health and supporting healing.

HOW THIS COOKBOOK CAN BE USEFUL

The goal of this Peptic Ulcer Diet Cookbook is to support people who are managing peptic ulcers by offering a variety of nourishing meal options that are easy on the stomach and promote healing and symptom relief. Each recipe is carefully crafted to be low in acidity and fat, avoiding common trigger foods that may worsen ulcer symptoms. The recipes are delicious and practical.

With the help of this cookbook, people can enjoy tasty meals that are simple to make and customized to meet their dietary requirements. The recipes feature foods like lean proteins, whole grains, and fresh fruits and vegetables that are well-known for their ability to soothe the stomach and support digestive health. Whether cooking breakfast, lunch, dinner, or snacks, there is something for every taste and dietary preference in this cookbook, which makes it easier for people to follow the suggested diet for managing peptic ulcers.

ADVICE ON HOW TO USE THIS COOKBOOK

To get the most out of this Peptic Ulcer Diet Cookbook, plan your meals ahead of time to make sure you have the ingredients on hand.

Before you start cooking, carefully read over each recipe, noting any modifications you might need to make based on dietary restrictions or personal preferences. When cooking, choose lighter cooking techniques like steaming, baking, or grilling instead of frying or using a lot of oil.

These pointers will help you make the most of the recipes in this cookbook and support your journey toward better digestive health. Try experimenting with different flavor combinations and ingredients to make meals interesting and enjoyable. Pay attention to portion sizes and avoid overeating, as large meals can put strain on the stomach and worsen ulcer symptoms. Stay hydrated throughout the day by drinking water or herbal teas, and limit intake of caffeinated or carbonated beverages.

FAQS & FREQUENTLY ASKED QUESTIONS

It is common to have questions and concerns about safe foods to eat and how to prepare gentle-on-the-tummy meals when managing peptic ulcers with dietary changes.

Examples of commonly asked questions are: should spicy foods be avoided completely (yes, they can exacerbate symptoms), is dairy suitable (low-fat options like yogurt can be beneficial), and Is herbal tea better than coffee (yes, as they are less acidic)?

This cookbook addresses these issues by offering concise guidelines and recipes that promote digestive health and overall well-being. Other common concerns include the role of stress in ulcer flare-ups, the effectiveness of dietary changes alone versus combined with medication, and how to handle occasional indulgences without harm. It's important to speak with a healthcare provider or a dietitian if you have specific dietary restrictions or medical conditions that may impact your ulcer management.

CHAPTER TWO

AN OVERVIEW OF PEPTIC ULCERS

HOW DO PEPTIC ULCERS OCCUR?

Peptic ulcers are painful sores that develop on the lining of the stomach, small intestine, or esophagus. They can be caused by an imbalance between the digestive fluids in the stomach and the protective mucosal layer that lines these organs. The most common type of ulcer is gastric ulcer, which occurs in the stomach, while duodenal ulcers develop in the upper part of the small intestine. The bacterium Helicobacter pylori (H. pylori) or long-term use of NSAIDs like aspirin or ibuprofen are the usual causes of ulcers, though stress and spicy foods can exacerbate their symptoms.

PEPTIC ULCER CAUSES

The main cause of peptic ulcers is an imbalance between the digestive enzyme pepsin, stomach acid, and the protective mucosal lining of the stomach and intestines. Another risk factor is infection with Helicobacter pylori (H. pylori), which weakens the protective qualities of the mucosal layer, allowing stomach acid to damage the underlying tissue. Long-term use of nonsteroidal anti-inflammatory drugs (NSAIDs) like aspirin, ibuprofen, and naproxen can also cause ulcers by irritating the stomach lining and decreasing its capacity to withstand acid exposure. Other risk factors include excessive alcohol consumption, smoking, and stress, but they do not directly cause ulcers.

SIGNS AND PROGNOSIS

Peptic ulcer symptoms can vary, but they usually involve a burning or painful feeling in the stomach area, especially after meals or at night. Other symptoms that may occur are bloating, heartburn, nausea, and vomiting. Severe ulcers can lead to complications like bleeding or perforation, which need to be treated right away. A combination of medical history, physical examination, and diagnostic tests are usually used to make the diagnosis. Endoscopy is a common procedure that involves inserting a flexible tube with a camera through the mouth to examine the esophagus, stomach, and duodenum for ulcers. During endoscopy, biopsies may be taken to check for H. pylori infection or rule out other conditions. Imaging tests, such as X-rays or CT scans, may be used if complications like bleeding or perforation ar.

PEPTIC ULCER TYPES

The location and underlying causes of peptic ulcers are classified as follows: gastric ulcers develop in the lining of the stomach, whereas duodenal ulcers develop in the upper part of the small intestine, known as the duodenum; gastric ulcers are more likely to be associated with NSAID use and H. pylori infection, while duodenal ulcers are primarily linked to H. pylori infection; once thought to be major contributors, stress and spicy foods are now recognized as factors that can exacerbate symptoms rather than directly cause ulcers; the symptoms and treatment strategy may differ slightly depending on the type and location of ulcers; however, both types are treated similarly with medications to reduce stomach acid production, antibiotics to eradicate H. pylori infection, and lifestyle modifications to alla.

DIET IS IMPORTANT FOR TREATMENT

A peptic ulcer diet usually emphasizes foods that do not increase stomach acid production or irritate the stomach lining. This includes eating more often and in smaller portions to reduce stomach acid secretion and avoiding spicy foods, coffee, alcohol, and acidic beverages like citrus juices. Instead, the diet focuses on incorporating whole grains, lean proteins, fruits, and vegetables that are easy to digest and promote healing. Certain foods, like probiotics-rich yogurt and foods high in fiber, may help to support digestive health and reduce inflammation.

CHAPTER THREE

FUNDAMENTALS OF A DIET FOR PEPTIC ULCERS

OBJECTIVES OF THE DIET

A peptic ulcer diet focuses on keeping the balance of nutrients to support overall health and well-being during the healing process, as well as managing symptoms and promoting healing of the ulcerated areas in the stomach or duodenum. This includes minimizing irritation and allowing the ulcer to heal by reducing stomach acid production. The diet achieves this by emphasizing foods that are gentle on the digestive system and less likely to stimulate acid production.

To accomplish these ends, the diet usually consists of low-fat and low-acidity foods, since these can exacerbate ulcer symptoms. It also promotes the consumption of foods that offer vital nutrients, like vitamins A, C, and E, which are critical for tissue repair. People who follow this diet may be able to lessen discomfort, avoid complications, and aid in the healing of tissues that have been ulcerated. Speaking with a healthcare provider is necessary to customize the diet to each patient's needs and track their progress.

FOODS TO ADD

Foods that are low in acidity and fat, like non-citrus fruits like apples and bananas, vegetables like carrots and spinach, and lean proteins like skinless chicken and fish, are essential components of a peptic ulcer diet. Whole grains like oats and brown rice also provide fiber and can help regulate digestion without irritating the stomach.

Dairy products should be low-fat or fat-free to prevent consuming too much fat; healthier fats from nuts and olive oil can also be helpful in moderation; herbal teas and non-acidic juices, such as watermelon or pear juice, can hydrate without making ulcer symptoms worse; by incorporating these foods into their diet, people with peptic ulcers can effectively lessen discomfort and support the healing process.

FOOD TO AVOID

A peptic ulcer diet must exclude certain foods to prevent flare-ups and to aid in the healing process. Citrus fruits and juices, tomatoes, vinegar, and high-acid foods can aggravate ulcers by raising stomach acidity; hot sauces, chili peppers, black pepper, and other seasonings can also aggravate symptoms by inducing discomfort and promoting acid production.

Avoiding or reducing the consumption of fatty and fried foods can help people manage their peptic ulcers and promote healing. Limiting the consumption of caffeine-containing beverages such as coffee, tea, and cola can also help people secrete less acid. Finally, reducing or eliminating alcohol and carbonated drinks can help people's stomach lining become inflamed and slow down the healing process.

TIPS FOR MEAL PLANNING

To ensure that they meet their nutritional needs while minimizing symptoms, people on a peptic ulcer diet must effectively plan their meals. Eating smaller, more frequent meals throughout the day is preferable to large meals, which can put additional strain on the digestive system. Each meal should contain a variety of foods from all food groups to ensure a balanced intake of nutrients.

A food diary can help track triggers and identify which foods worsen symptoms, allowing for better diet management.

Steaming, baking, or grilling instead of frying reduces fat content and makes foods easier to digest. Including fiber-rich foods like fruits, vegetables, and whole grains supports healthy digestion and can help regulate bowel movements.

ESSENTIALS FOR THE PANTRY AND SHOPPING

Stocking up on pantry staples that support the suggested food choices is crucial when following a peptic ulcer diet. Whole grains, like oats, brown rice, and whole wheat pasta, offer fiber and vital nutrients without upsetting the stomach, and lean proteins, like skinless chicken, fish, and beans, are easier to digest and aid in muscle growth and repair.

Select low-fat or fat-free dairy products, such as milk and yogurt, to minimize fat consumption while obtaining necessary calcium and vitamin D. Low-acid fruits, like apples, bananas, and pears, offer vitamins and minerals that promote general health. Low-acid vegetables, like broccoli, spinach, and carrots, are easy on the stomach and high in antioxidants that can promote healing.

A well-rounded peptic ulcer diet that effectively promotes healing and reduces discomfort can be maintained by stocking essential pantry items like herbal teas, non-acidic juices (like pear or watermelon juice), nuts, and olive oil in moderation. Healthy fats like olive oil and nuts can support heart health and overall well-being.

CHAPTER FOUR

MEAL PLANNING AND PREPARATION

WEEKLY MEAL PLANNING SCHEDULE

Weekly meal planning will make your peptic ulcer diet regimen much easier to follow. Begin by figuring out what nutrient-dense, ulcer-friendly foods you like and that are easy on your stomach. Try to include a range of lean proteins, like chicken, fish, and tofu, as they are easier to digest. Add high-fiber fruits and vegetables, preferably well-cooked or blended to help with digestion. Whole grains, like brown rice and oats, can offer important nutrients without irritating your stomach lining.

Partition your weekly meal plan into digestible chunks, concentrating on breakfast, lunch, dinner, and snacks. You may also want to think about preparing ingredients that are versatile, like cooked grains, steamed vegetables, and boiled eggs, ahead of time. This will help you put together meals quickly throughout the week, cutting down on prep time and guaranteeing diet consistency. Portion control will help you prevent overindulging, which can aggravate symptoms. Finally, keep a range of ulcer-safe snacks on hand, such as yogurt, almonds, and smoothies, to sustain your energy levels in between meals.

Meal plans should be modified by your symptoms and nutritional requirements; you should also keep an eye on how your body reacts to various foods and make necessary adjustments to preserve digestive comfort. With careful planning and mindful eating, you can successfully manage your peptic ulcer diet and still enjoy satisfying, flavorful meals.

STRATEGIES FOR BATCH COOKING

Making large batches of these ingredients ahead of time and storing them in portion-sized containers for easy and quick meals is a practical way to make sure you have ulcer-friendly meals available every day of the week. Start by choosing recipes that fit your dietary restrictions and emphasize simplicity and nutrient density. Select easy-to-digest ingredients like cooked vegetables, lean proteins, and whole grains.

Opt for more gentle cooking techniques such as baking, steaming, or boiling instead of frying or grilling. Add flavorings such as herbs and spices without adding extra fat or acidity, which can aggravate ulcer symptoms. When preparing meals in bulk, give priority to items that can be eaten cold or reheated with ease.

Create a weekly batch cooking schedule to help you stick to your peptic ulcer diet. Set aside a day to prepare meals, spending time cooking and portioning food for the next few days.

Label and store your cooked meals in the freezer or refrigerator to keep them fresh and easily accessible. By implementing batch cooking techniques, you can keep your diet consistent, reduce the stress that comes with meal planning, and promote digestive health.

ADVICE FOR DINING OUT

Eating out requires careful thought and preparation when on a peptic ulcer diet. Start by looking for restaurants that have menu items that fit your dietary requirements; these should emphasize simple, fresh ingredients and provide dishes that can be customized to meet your needs. Before you go, check the menu online or give them a call to see if there are any ingredient substitutions or modifications available.

Select dishes that are grilled, baked, or steamed rather than fried or spicy, as these can exacerbate symptoms of ulcers. Ask for sauces and dressings to be served on the side to manage portion sizes and prevent too much fat or acidity. Steamed vegetables, baked potatoes, or rice are good side orders because they are easy on the stomach and contain important nutrients.

By following these tips, you can enjoy dining out while following your peptic ulcer diet, promoting digestive comfort and overall well-being. Pace yourself during meals and chew thoroughly to aid in digestion.

Avoid alcohol and caffeinated beverages, as they can irritate the stomach lining. Think about dining during off-peak hours to reduce stress and ensure attentive service.

RECIPES FOR OPTIMAL DIGESTIVE HEALTH

Choosing lean cuts of meat and poultry and removing visible fat and skin before cooking will reduce acidity and fat content. Gentle cooking techniques are crucial for maintaining digestive health when following a diet for peptic ulcers. Start by steaming or boiling vegetables to soften their texture and enhance digestibility. These methods preserve nutrients while minimizing the risk of irritating the stomach lining.

Add anti-inflammatory and digestive herbs and spices like ginger, turmeric, and basil. Sauté and stir-fry in small amounts of olive oil or vegetable broth; steer clear of high heat and long cooking times. Slow cooking techniques like braising or simmering help to soften tough meats and improve flavor without sacrificing nutritional value.

Try pureeing or blending ingredients to make easier-to-digest soups, sauces, and dips. Focus on whole grains, such as quinoa, oats, and barley, as they are high in fiber and help maintain regular digestion. Once you have mastered these cooking methods, you will be able to make delicious, nutrient-dense, and nutrient-rich meals that will support digestive health and fit into your peptic ulcer diet.

EASY COOKING USING KITCHEN TOOLS

Having the right appliances in your kitchen can help you achieve your peptic ulcer diet goals and make meal preparation easier. A good blender or food processor can be used to puree fruits, vegetables, and grains into smooth, stomach-friendly textures. A steamer basket or microwave steamer can be used to quickly and effectively cook vegetables without using too much heat or oil.

Select nonstick cookware to cut down on the amount of cooking oil you use and the fat in your food. Keep measuring cups and spoons in your pantry to help you portion ingredients correctly and maintain diet consistency. Use a sharp chef's knife and cutting board to cut up fruits, vegetables, and meats precisely.

Invest in kitchen tools like a garlic press or citrus juicer to easily add fresh flavors to your food. Have a variety of storage containers of different sizes on hand to arrange and store cooked meals and ingredients. With these kitchen tools, you can prepare meals more quickly, keep your diet consistent, and consume wholesome meals that promote comfort in your digestive system.

RECIPES FOR BREAKFAST

HEALTHY DRINKS

Fruits like bananas, mangoes, or spinach make a base for a nutritious smoothie; add a variety of fruits like berries, bananas, or kale for natural sweetness and a dose of vitamins; and add ingredients like Greek yogurt, almond milk, or protein powder for extra protein. Nutritious smoothies are a great way to start your day with a boost of vitamins and minerals, and they can be customized based on your dietary preferences and nutritional needs.

Superfoods such as chia seeds, flaxseeds, or spirulina can be added to improve both the flavor and nutritional value.

These ingredients not only add texture but also provide healthy fats and essential nutrients. Blend everything until smooth, adding extra liquid or water as needed to adjust the consistency. Healthy smoothies are a great option for on-the-go or sit-down breakfasts, and they are especially good for people who have peptic ulcers because they are easy on the stomach and provide essential nutrients without causing discomfort.

FIBER-PACKED OATMEAL CONVERSIONS

A traditional breakfast option, oatmeal can be enhanced in nutritional value by adding additional fiber-rich ingredients. To begin, cook rolled oats (a good source of soluble fiber known to support digestive health) in water or milk until creamy. Next, add different toppings to your oatmeal to add extra fiber: add fruits (bananas, apples, or berries) for sweetness and extra nutrients; add ground flaxseeds, chia seeds, or nuts (almonds or walnuts) to increase the amount of fiber in your oatmeal.

When it comes to oatmeal, variations with low-acid fruits and nuts can be calming and filling for those on a peptic ulcer diet. Try varying the flavor profile by adding cinnamon, vanilla extract, or a small amount of honey for sweetness. Oatmeal which is high in fiber is a great breakfast option for people who are managing peptic ulcers because it helps regulate blood sugar levels and makes you feel full.

WHOLESOME EGG RECIPES

Eggs are a nutrient-dense, adaptable ingredient that can be used in a variety of healthful breakfast dishes. They are full and satisfying for breakfast, and when following a peptic ulcer diet, eggs should be prepared in a way that is gentle on the stomach. For example, scrambled eggs cooked in a nonstick pan with a little olive oil or butter are easy to digest and go well with whole-grain toast or steamed vegetables.

Eggs can be enjoyed in moderation as part of a peptic ulcer diet, providing essential nutrients without aggravating symptoms. Experiment with different cooking methods and ingredients to create flavorful and nourishing egg dishes that support digestive health. As an alternative, try making a vegetable omelet with spinach, bell peppers, and mushrooms for added fiber and nutrients. Poached eggs served on whole-grain English muffins with avocado or smoked salmon can provide a balanced breakfast rich in healthy fats and protein.

LOW-ACID FRUIT SELECTIONS

Fruits that are low in acidity are better for people with peptic ulcers because acidic fruits can aggravate the lining of the stomach.

Fruits that are low in acidity include bananas, melons, and pears, which are generally well-tolerated by most people and contain vitamins, minerals, and natural sugars without causing discomfort or acid reflux. You can enjoy low-acid fruits fresh, sliced over yogurt or oatmeal, or blended into smoothies.

Choosing low-acid fruit options can help you enjoy a delicious breakfast that supports digestive health and helps manage symptoms of peptic ulcers. Make a fruit salad with a variety of low-acid fruits like apples, grapes, and kiwi. Sprinkle with a squeeze of lemon juice or a drizzle of honey for added flavor. Another idea is to blend low-acid fruits into homemade fruit sorbets or popsicles using natural sweeteners like agave syrup or maple syrup.

IDEAS FOR QUICK AND SIMPLE BREAKFASTS

In a hurry? Here are some quick and simple breakfast ideas that can still be satisfying and nutritious—especially for people with peptic ulcers. To make overnight oats, soak rolled oats in milk or yogurt overnight, then top with fruits, nuts, and honey in the morning.

Greek yogurt with honey and a few nuts is a healthy and protein-rich breakfast that is also gentle on the stomach. For a savory twist, spread avocado or almond butter on whole-grain toast and top with chia seeds for extra nutrition.

These quick and simple breakfast ideas ensure that people with peptic ulcers can start their day with nourishing meals that are easy to prepare and gentle on the stomach. Smoothies made with low-acid fruits, spinach, and a scoop of protein powder can be blended in minutes and enjoyed on the go. For a balanced meal, consider making a quinoa salad with diced vegetables and a light vinaigrette dressing. Quinoa is a nutrient-dense grain that provides protein and fiber, supporting digestive health without aggravating symptoms.

RECIPES FOR LUNCH

LIGHT DRESSINGS AND SALADS

A peptic ulcer diet must include light salads because they provide a nutrient-dense, hydrating choice without aggravating symptoms. Start with a base of mildly acidic leafy greens, such as romaine lettuce or spinach, and add colorful vegetables, like bell peppers, cucumbers, and cherry tomatoes, for extra flavor and nutrients. To further improve the salad's flavor, try adding low-fat, easily digested lean proteins, like tofu or grilled chicken breast.

For dressings, try light vinaigrettes made with olive oil and vinegar; stay away from creamy or highly acidic dressings as they can irritate the lining of the stomach. To make a basic dressing, combine olive oil, balsamic vinegar, Dijon mustard, and a small amount of salt and pepper; this adds flavor without sacrificing health. To add some crunch and healthy fats, sprinkle some nuts or seeds over your salad; this adds texture and extra nutrients that are good for managing ulcers.

OPTIONS FOR LEAN PROTEIN

Lean meats, such as skinless poultry (such as chicken or turkey) and lean cuts of beef or pork, are excellent choices because they have less fat, which helps reduce the risk of irritation to the stomach lining.

For plant-based eaters, tofu, tempeh, and legumes like lentils and chickpeas provide plenty of protein without added fat. They are also high in fiber, which helps to maintain digestive health and effectively manage ulcer symptoms.

Instead of frying, when cooking lean proteins, use techniques like grilling, baking, or steaming, which use less added fat and oil and result in a healthier meal; season your proteins with herbs and spices rather than thick sauces, which can be hard on the stomach; and combine these lean protein options into salads or main dishes to make filling, healing, and overall well-being meals.

WHOLE GRAIN SELECTIONS

A peptic ulcer diet must include whole grains because they contain complex carbohydrates and fiber that support digestive health and provide sustained energy. Whole grains, such as brown rice, quinoa, whole wheat pasta, and oats, are less likely to irritate the stomach than refined grains and are high in fiber, which is important for regulating bowel movements and digestion.

Experiment with different whole-grain options to find dishes that you enjoy and that are gentle on your stomach. When incorporating whole grains into your meals, try recipes like whole wheat pasta dishes with vegetables and lean proteins, whole grain salads, or stir-fries with brown rice. These dishes provide a balanced combination of nutrients and flavors while supporting ulcer healing. Steer clear of heavily processed grains and white flour products because they have a high glycemic index and can aggravate ulcer symptoms.

VEGETABLE-BASED RECIPES

Due to their high nutrient density and fiber content, vegetables are crucial to a diet for peptic ulcers because they support overall health and digestive health. When choosing vegetables, choose non-acidic ones like leafy greens (kale, spinach), root vegetables (carrots, sweet potatoes), and cruciferous vegetables (broccoli, cauliflower). These vegetables are full of antioxidants, vitamins, and minerals that help heal and reduce inflammation in the stomach lining.

Vegetable-centric dishes benefit from cooking techniques such as steaming, roasting, or sautéing with little to no oil to retain their nutritional value and facilitate digestion. Be wary of overly spicy or highly seasoned vegetables, as they can cause upset stomachs. Use a range of vibrant vegetables in soups, stews, stir-fries, or as side dishes to main courses to ensure a varied intake of nutrients while maintaining an interesting and pleasurable mealtime experience.

IDEAS FOR CARRYING LUNCH ON THE GO

For people with peptic ulcers who require quick and simple meals to eat on the go, portable lunch ideas are crucial. Try whole grain wraps or sandwiches with lean proteins like turkey or grilled chicken, along with non-acidic vegetables and a light spread like avocado or hummus. These options are gentle on the stomach and offer a balanced mix of carbohydrates, protein, and fiber.

Alternatively, you could pack fruits like berries or apples for extra fiber and natural sweetness, or you could pack grain-based salads like quinoa or couscous salads mixed with vegetables and a light vinaigrette dressing. These salads are filling, nutrient-dense, and portable. Pick ingredients like mixed greens, cherry tomatoes, cucumber slices, and lean protein sources like boiled eggs or grilled tofu.

For snacks, choose low-acid yogurt with probiotics added for digestive health, or whole-grain crackers with cheese or nut butter.

RECIPES FOR DINNER

DELICIOUS FISH AND SHELLFISH

For example, a peptic ulcer diet cookbook featuring tasty fish and seafood dishes should emphasize options that are high in flavor but low in acidity. One way to achieve this is by selecting fish types such as salmon, which is high in omega-3 fatty acids and has anti-inflammatory qualities. A straightforward but tasty recipe would be to bake salmon fillets with a light lemon and herb seasoning, which would make it easy to digest while maintaining a satisfying flavor.

Shrimp is a very flexible seafood option. For example, you can sauté shrimp in olive oil and garlic, then toss them with whole-grain pasta and fresh tomatoes for a satisfying meal that is easy on the stomach. These dishes not only satisfy dietary requirements related to the treatment of peptic ulcers, but they also strike a balance between flavor and digestibility.

ENTREES WITH LEAN MEAT

A peptic ulcer diet cookbook should feature lean meat entrees that are low in fat and easy to digest. One way to prepare chicken breast is to grill or bake it with a light marinade of herbs and spices. This will keep the chicken breast flavorful and tender without adding to discomfort. Serving it with steamed vegetables or a small portion of brown rice makes for a balanced meal that promotes digestive health.

Lean pork or turkey cuts can also be added for variety. For example, roasting turkey tenderloin with seasonal vegetables makes a filling meal that is high in protein and important nutrients.

These recipes not only meet dietary requirements but also offer a range of options for people on a diet that prevents ulcers from occurring, making sure that meals are tasty and nutritious without sacrificing flavor.

MAIN COURSES FOR VEGETARIANS

An array of vibrant veggies, such as bell peppers, carrots, and broccoli, can be sautéed in olive oil and seasoned with herbs to create a hearty and nutritious stir-fry. Tofu or chickpeas can be added for protein. Vegetarian main courses in a peptic ulcer diet cookbook emphasize plant-based options that are gentle on the stomach but flavorful.

A lentil stew cooked with tomatoes, spinach, and flavorful spices like coriander and cumin would be an additional choice.

This dish is high in fiber and protein and also helps with digestive health because it has a comforting and easily digested flavor combination. These vegetarian recipes suit a variety of dietary needs and guarantee that the meals are appropriate for people who are treating peptic ulcers, which promotes overall wellness.

ASSORTMENTS AND SIDE DISHES

A peptic ulcer diet cookbook should have side dishes and accompaniments that go well with main courses and are easy on the stomach. For example, steamed veggies like carrots or green beans seasoned with a little olive oil and fresh herbs offer vitamins and minerals that are necessary without being uncomfortable, or a quinoa salad mixed with cucumbers, tomatoes, and a light vinaigrette is a cool and nourishing side dish.

When a person is in the mood for something heartier, mashed sweet potatoes flavored with a dash of cinnamon can be a cozy side dish to go with lean meat or vegetarian dishes.

These side dishes not only boost the nutritional content of meals but also support a balanced diet that promotes digestive health. People who make these choices can eat delicious meals while effectively managing their dietary needs.

ONE-POT DINNER IDEAS

One-pot dinner ideas are a great way to cut down on cooking time without sacrificing flavor or digestibility. Take a chicken and vegetable stew, for instance, which is made by simmering chicken thighs, potatoes, carrots, and celery in a flavorful broth flavored with herbs. This filling dish not only provides plenty of protein and nutrients but also reduces the amount of preparation and cleanup that is required.

Instead, a Mediterranean-inspired seafood paella with shrimp, mussels, and aromatic rice cooked in a tomato-based broth provides a filling and healthy alternative. These one-pot meals satisfy peptic ulcer dietary restrictions while providing a range of flavors and textures; by including these recipes in a peptic ulcer diet cookbook, people can enjoy healthful meals without sacrificing taste or health benefits.

RECIPES FOR SNACKS AND DESSERTS

HEALTHY SNACK SUGGESTIONS

Snacks are vital for sustaining energy levels and promoting general health, particularly for individuals on a peptic ulcer diet. It is important to choose high-nutrient, low-absorption snacks that are also gentle on the stomach. For example, sliced apples with a small dollop of almond butter are a healthy snack that provides fiber and good fats without making stomach problems worse. A handful of mixed nuts and seeds is a great snack that provides a balanced amount of protein and important minerals. These snacks are portable and can be made ahead of time, making them ideal for hectic schedules.

For a more savory option, try whole-grain crackers with a slice of low-fat cheese or hummus; the fiber from the whole grains helps with digestion, and the protein from the cheese or hummus provides satiety. Vegetable sticks, such as carrots, cucumbers, and bell peppers, dipped in a light dip, can be a refreshing and nutrient-dense snack that satisfies hunger while also supporting a balanced diet, which is essential for effectively managing symptoms of peptic ulcers.

Snackies that are too spicy, fried, or heavy in saturated fats should be avoided as they might worsen symptoms of ulcers; instead, look for satisfying but mildly inflammatory snacks that support general health and ease of digestion.

YOGURT AND FRESH FRUIT PARFAITS

For those on a peptic ulcer diet, fresh fruit and yogurt parfaits are a tasty and nourishing option. To begin, layer plain, unsweetened yogurt with fresh berries or diced fruits such as bananas, strawberries, or blueberries. Fruits provide vital vitamins and antioxidants, and yogurt offers probiotics that support gut health. To add some crunch and nutrition, sprinkle chopped nuts or granola between the layers.

Aim for harmony between textures and flavors when assembling the parfait.

The tartness of the yogurt contrasts with the juicy fruits, making for a filling snack or light dinner. This combination tastes great and offers a good balance of carbohydrates, proteins, and fats to support stable blood sugar levels and digestive comfort.

Fresh fruit and yogurt parfaits are a flexible and nutrient-dense addition to a peptic ulcer diet plan. Try experimenting with different fruits and toppings based on personal preferences and seasonal availability. To customize your parfait, consider using Greek yogurt for extra protein or adding a drizzle of honey for sweetness.

LOW-CARB BAKED GOODS

For those who are managing the symptoms of a peptic ulcer, low-fat baked goods can be a reassuring and fulfilling option. When baking, look for recipes that call for whole wheat flour or oats, which offer fiber and nutrients without upsetting the stomach. You can also bake muffins using mashed bananas or unsweetened applesauce instead of oil or butter, which lowers the fat content while adding natural sweetness and moisture.

For a savory twist, try baking whole-wheat crackers or flatbreads seasoned with herbs and spices for added flavor. Another option is to bake whole-grain bread or rolls using small amounts of healthy fats like olive oil or avocado oil. These baked goods offer complex carbohydrates that provide sustained energy without spiking blood sugar levels.

Portion control is key when consuming low-fat baked goods to prevent discomfort from overindulging. Combine these treats with a small portion of fruits or vegetables or a source of lean protein to make a well-balanced snack or meal. Low-fat baked goods can be a tasty addition to a peptic ulcer diet plan if you use healthy ingredients and baking techniques.

SWEETS WITH VERY LITTLE SUGAR

A peptic ulcer diet allows you to enjoy sweets with little sugar, as long as you stick to foods that are easy on the stomach and satisfy your cravings. Fruit-based desserts, such as baked pears or apples with cinnamon on top, are a great way to get natural sweetness and fiber without adding extra sugar to your diet. You can even bake these until they are soft for a warm, comforting treat.

Alternatively, make your fruit sorbet at home with frozen fruit blended with a tiny bit of yogurt or coconut milk. This is a low-sugar, refreshing dessert that can be made with any fruit, including berries, mangoes, or pineapple. If you want to go all out, top it with chopped nuts or seeds for extra texture and nutrients.

Sweet treats can be occasionally enjoyed as part of a balanced peptic ulcer diet, promoting satisfaction without compromising digestive health. When selecting sweet treats, choose recipes that use natural sweeteners like honey or maple syrup in moderation, avoiding refined sugars that can irritate the stomach lining.

TIPS FOR HEALTHY SNACKING

Maintaining energy levels and promoting digestive health—especially for individuals with peptic ulcers—requires incorporating healthy snacking habits.

To start, schedule snacks in advance and keep wholesome options on hand, like pre-cut fruits and vegetables stored in portioned containers. This will prevent you from reaching for unhealthy snacks when you're hungry.

A balanced combination of macronutrients can help stabilize blood sugar levels throughout the day. For example, snack on a handful of almonds or walnuts with a piece of fruit, or enjoy a small serving of plain yogurt with fresh berries. These high-fiber and high-protein snacks can promote satiety and aid indigestion.

Aim for easy-to-digest snacks that are low in fat, especially saturated and trans fats, which can aggravate ulcer symptoms. By incorporating these healthy snacking tips into daily routines, people can support overall well-being and effectively manage the symptoms of peptic ulcers. When snacking, be mindful of portion sizes to prevent overeating, which can lead to discomfort.

DRINKS AND SMOOTHIES

OPTIONS FOR HYDRATING DRINKS

To help manage peptic ulcers, it's important to drink enough water, herbal teas, and diluted fruit juices. Herbal teas, like chamomile or ginger, have soothing properties that can calm digestive discomfort. They are caffeine-free and can be enjoyed hot or cold, making them versatile options throughout the day. Water is the ultimate hydrator, helping to maintain mucosal integrity and aid digestion. Aim for at least 8 glasses daily, adjusting based on your activity level and climate.

Fruit juices: Choose low-acid varieties, such as apple or pear juice, and dilute them with water to lessen their irritating effect on the lining of the stomach. Another great option is coconut water, which is naturally electrolyte-rich and helps hydrate without added sugars or artificial additives. Including these hydrating beverages in your daily routine will help you stay hydrated overall as well as manage the symptoms of peptic ulcers and maintain digestive health.

RECIPES FOR ANTI-INFLAMMATORY SMOOTHIES

Smoothies that reduce inflammation and soothe the digestive tract are a delicious way to support healing from peptic ulcers. A base of gentle-on-the-tummy non-citrus fruits, like bananas, berries, or mangoes, should be added, followed by leafy greens like spinach or kale, which are rich in fiber and antioxidants, promoting gut health, and a source of healthy fats, like avocado or flaxseed oil, to improve nutrient absorption and satiety.

Use a non-dairy milk alternative such as almond milk or coconut milk as the liquid base to avoid dairy-related discomfort for some people. Blend these ingredients until smooth, adjusting consistency with water or ice as desired. Enjoy these smoothies as a nutrient-dense snack or meal replacement to support healing and alleviate symptoms associated with peptic ulcers. Turmeric, known for its curcumin content, has potent anti-inflammatory properties. Fresh ginger can also be beneficial for soothing stomach irritation and aiding digestion.

HERBAL INFUSIONS AND TEAS

Herbal teas and infusions are a great way to support digestive health and ease the symptoms of peptic ulcers. Some of the well-known benefits of herbal teas include chamomile, which reduces stomach acidity and promotes relaxation; peppermint, which soothes the digestive tract and helps relieve gas and bloating; and slippery elm, which coats the stomach lining to protect it from irritation and promote healing.

Herbal infusions like marshmallow root or licorice root can also be helpful for their mucilaginous qualities, which soothe and protect the stomach lining. Choose caffeine-free varieties to avoid stimulating acid production, and when possible, opt for organic or sustainably sourced herbs to ensure purity and effectiveness. Including these herbal teas and infusions into your daily routine can offer natural relief and support healing from peptic ulcers. Fresh herbs like basil or fennel can be used to make teas that can help with digestion and reduce inflammation.

A LOOK AT COFFEE AND CAFFEINE

For people who have peptic ulcers, controlling caffeine and coffee intake is crucial because these substances can exacerbate symptoms and increase the production of stomach acid. If you like coffee, choose low-acid or cold brew varieties, as these are less likely to irritate your stomach; reduce the strength or caffeine content by blending regular coffee with decaffeinated options; and stay away from acidic flavorings like citrus or espresso shots, which can be more concentrated and acidic.

Green tea and herbal teas are two alternative caffeine sources that can be mildly more gentle on the stomach while still offering a slight energy boost.

Pay attention to how your body reacts to caffeine and modify your intake to effectively manage symptoms. Try different brewing methods and preparation techniques to see what works best for your digestive health while still getting the benefits of caffeine in moderation.

THE EFFECTS OF ALCOHOL

For people who are managing peptic ulcers, it is recommended to limit or avoid alcohol consumption. If you do choose to drink, go for light or non-alcoholic options like mocktails or alcohol-free beer and wine options. These can provide a social drink without hurting digestive health. Alcohol can exacerbate symptoms of peptic ulcers by increasing stomach acid production and irritating the digestive tract.

To support healing and effectively manage symptoms, moderation is key when it comes to alcohol consumption. Limit intake to one drink per day for women and up to two drinks per day for men. Avoid mixing alcohol with medications used to treat peptic ulcers as this may interfere with their effectiveness or exacerbate side effects. Listen to your body and prioritize its needs when making decisions about alcohol consumption.

CHAPTER FIVE

RECIPES FOR SPECIAL OCCASIONS AND HOLIDAYS

IDEAS FOR HOLIDAY MEALS

To prepare holiday meals that are both delicious and easy on the stomach cooks with peptic ulcers should take special care to select foods that are low in fat and acidity, as these factors can aggravate the symptoms of the ulcer. Lean proteins, such as chicken or turkey, are a good choice, and there should be an abundance of fresh produce, especially leafy greens, root vegetables, and non-citrus fruits.

Main course ideas include baked salmon with a light lemon and herb sauce or roasted turkey breast seasoned with mild herbs. For sides, try quinoa salad with cucumber and mint, roasted sweet potatoes, or steamed green beans with a little olive oil. Desserts can be tricky, but fruit-based options like honey-baked apples or baked apples with cinnamon can provide a sweet finish without upsetting the stomach.

INGREDIENTS THAT ARE IN SEASON

Seasonal foods can provide diversity and freshness to a diet for peptic ulcers while also promoting digestive health. In the spring and summer, eat a lot of fresh produce, especially leafy greens, berries, and melons, which are easy on the stomach and can be eaten raw or cooked just enough to retain their nutrients and soft texture.

Root vegetables, such as sweet potatoes, carrots, and squash, come into season in the fall and winter and make for a wholesome and satisfying side dish when roasted or mashed. In the cooler months, apples and pears are also in season and make for a calming dessert when baked or stewed with spices like nutmeg and cinnamon.

TIPS FOR GUESTS WITH PEPTIC ULCERS

When you host with a peptic ulcer, you need to make sure that everyone has a good time and that you are well too.

Let them know about your dietary restrictions so they can make accommodations or offer other options. You can also serve food buffet-style so that people can help themselves to whatever they want and you can maintain control over portion sizes and menu selections.

Make sure to serve light, easily digestible food; steer clear of spicy, acidic, or fatty foods that may exacerbate symptoms. Provide a range of options, such as salads and cooked vegetables, as well as lean proteins like grilled chicken or fish. Offer non-alcoholic beverage options, such as herbal teas, infused waters, and mocktails, to stay hydrated and comfortable during the event.

MODIFYING RECIPES FOR EVENTS

When you have a peptic ulcer, you can modify recipes for parties in a way that makes them both stomach-friendly and enjoyable for all attendees. For example, you can replace acidic ingredients like tomatoes in pasta sauces or casseroles with milder options like roasted bell peppers, and you can add flavor to food without irritating your stomach by using herbs and spices like ginger, basil, and oregano.

Adjust cooking techniques to lower fat content by baking, grilling, or steaming instead of frying. In dessert recipes, swap out heavy creams for yogurt or coconut milk to achieve creamy textures without making your stomach churn. Make as much of your preparations ahead of time to cut down on stress and give yourself time to make any necessary adjustments.

CHAPTER SIX

TIPS FOR STRESS MANAGEMENT AND LIFESTYLE

STRESS MANAGEMENT'S SIGNIFICANCE

Adopting effective stress management techniques is essential for symptom relief and healing. Stress management plays a crucial role in managing peptic ulcers by reducing the physiological responses that can exacerbate symptoms. Stress causes the body to release hormones like cortisol and adrenaline, which can increase stomach acid production and decrease blood flow to the digestive system, potentially worsening ulcer symptoms.

By focusing attention on the present moment, mindfulness meditation is a useful technique that helps people become more aware of their thoughts and feelings without passing judgment. Progressive muscle relaxation is another helpful technique that helps people reduce stress by systematically tensing and relaxing different muscle groups.

This method not only helps people reduce stress immediately but also helps them manage their ulcers over the long term by reducing stress-related exacerbations.

Apart from specific relaxation methods, lifestyle changes like prioritizing and managing time can also help lower stress levels. People who organize their tasks and set realistic goals feel more in control of their daily lives, which lowers stress levels overall. Hobbies and outdoor activities can also help people feel better emotionally and improve their general well-being, which can help manage peptic ulcers more healthily.

TECHNIQUES FOR RELAXATION

Deep breathing exercises, like diaphragmatic breathing, involve slow, deep inhalations and exhalations that activate the body's relaxation response. This technique reduces heart rate and promotes feelings of calmness, making it an accessible and effective stress management tool.

Several relaxation techniques can help with stress management, which is crucial for alleviating peptic ulcer symptoms and promoting healing.

Another technique is progressive muscle relaxation (PMR), which involves systematically tensing and relaxing muscle groups throughout the body. Guided imagery, which involves visualizing peaceful scenes or positive outcomes, can also induce relaxation by refocusing attention away from stressors and promoting mental clarity. By releasing physical tension, PMR not only promotes relaxation but also helps individuals become more aware of their bodily responses to stress.

In addition, mind-body exercises such as yoga and tai chi are beneficial additions to a holistic approach to managing peptic ulcers because they combine physical movement with mindfulness and promote relaxation and stress reduction. People can develop resilience against stress and support their digestive health by incorporating these techniques into their daily routines.

EXERCISE FOR A HEALTHY DIGESTIVE SYSTEM

Physical activity stimulates the gastrointestinal tract, promoting more efficient digestion and nutrient absorption; it also helps regulate bowel movements, reducing the likelihood of constipation, which can exacerbate ulcer symptoms. Regular exercise is crucial for maintaining digestive health and managing peptic ulcers.

Aerobic exercises, like swimming, jogging, or walking, increase blood flow and oxygenation throughout the body, which benefits the digestive system and aids in the healing of ulcerated tissues. Exercises that are strength-training, like weightlifting or resistance banding, help to build muscle mass and support metabolic processes, which support improved digestive health.

In addition, exercise is essential for stress management because it triggers the release of endorphins, which are organic mood enhancers that lower stress and boost feelings of well-being.

People with peptic ulcers can effectively manage stress levels and enhance their quality of life by adding regular physical activity to their routines.

THE FUNCTION OF SLEEP

Good sleep is critical for the treatment and healing of peptic ulcers because it helps the body renew and repair damaged tissues, including ulcer-affected tissues. Enough sleep also boosts immunity, assisting the body in fending off infections that might impede the healing process.

Promoting restful sleep requires establishing a regular sleep schedule and developing a calming bedtime routine, which may involve actions like shutting off electronics, engaging in relaxation exercises like deep breathing or meditation, and making sure that the sleep environment is comfortable and free of distractions.

In addition, a balanced diet and avoiding large meals right before bed can help prevent discomfort and reflux symptoms that could interfere with sleep.

People can improve their quality of sleep and help their peptic ulcers heal by emphasizing sleep hygiene and treating any underlying sleep disorders.

MODIFICATIONS TO LIFESTYLE FOR EXTENDED WELL-BEING

Adopting healthy lifestyle adjustments is essential for long-term wellness and ulcer management, in addition to specific stress management techniques and physical activities. This includes limiting intake of spicy foods, caffeine, alcohol, and tobacco, and maintaining a balanced diet rich in fruits, vegetables, lean proteins, and whole grains.

Regular meals and snacks spaced throughout the day can prevent excessive stomach acid production and promote more stable blood sugar levels, which contribute to overall well-being.

Adequate water intake also helps maintain mucosal integrity and supports the protective lining of the stomach and intestines.

Additionally, timely management of ulcer symptoms and necessary plan modifications are ensured by routine medical check-ups and consultations with healthcare providers. Individuals can effectively manage peptic ulcers and enjoy improved quality of life by prioritizing self-care, stress management, and healthy lifestyle choices.

www.ingramcontent.com/pod-product-compliance
Lightning Source LLC
Chambersburg PA
CBHW072018230526
45479CB00008B/254